Prayers for
Nurses

By D. Duane Engler
& Marlene Graeve, RN

Galatians 6:2

"Carry each other's burdens, and in this way you will

fulfill the law of Christ."

Check out other titles by D. Duane Engler at Amazon.com

The Christian Revival Diet™ © 2013

Numerous Titles in the 40 Prayers™ Series © 2013 and the 40 Christian Prayers™ Series

40 by 40: 40 Short Stories with Less Than 40 Words © 2013

40 Prayers and Proverbs™

40 Prayers and Psalms™

Additional books in development.

If you are in the nursing profession, you may feel as if you have given away your last ounce of compassion.

The well-worn nursing path may be called burn-out, caregiver fatigue, weariness or downright discouragement. Whatever the verbiage, when the helter-skelter days are more the norm than the exception, nurses may come to the realization that they need help.

40 Prayers for Nurses is a cry for a companion to make sense of the happenings of our day. All the pieces can fall into place when our focus is on Jesus. He is the only one that can get us off the detour we have come to know as routine. To get on a straight path we need Jesus' promises and presence. The route is through prayer, using the Bible as a map. We recommend trying to pray these prayers over 40 days, taking notes and reflecting on How God's word has helped refresh your soul. We can be renewed by Christ's love, so we can once again, renew others.

Let's get to prayer!

To God be the glory,

Marlene Graeve, RN & D. Duane Engler

1

Not Growing Weary

Some days nursing seems more difficult than I ever expected. Sorrow, busyness, risk for errors and lawsuits, coworkers not working as a team, emesis, diarrhea, and wounds-the list can go on and on.
Still, there is nothing I would rather do!
Lord, walk beside me and do not allow me to grow weary and quit.
Give me strength and persistence.
In fact, I need all nine fruits of the Holy Spirit: love, joy, peace, patience, kindness, goodness, faithfulness, gentleness, and self-control.
Help me to be effective and make a difference in the life of at least one person.
If it is only one person in my entire career, and that is your will, I am willing to accept that.
I will keep my eyes open for the person You may be presenting today.

Galatians 6:9

"Let us not become weary in doing good, for at the proper time we will reap a harvest if we do not give up."

2

Love is the Law

Jesus, Your love is all that I need. Your love is the law. Help me obey Your
commands.
What I don't understand, please give me the clarity to see.
Show me the way!
Show me Your wisdom!
Show me everything I need to do!
I know the pain I'm experiencing in this life is to draw me closer to You.
Let me experience discomfort only for Your glory, Lord Jesus.
Help me to turn everything in my life towards You and learn to love like You do.

John 13:34-35

*"A new command I give you: Love one another. As I have loved you, so you must
love one another. By this everyone will know that you are my disciples, if you love
one another."*

3

Trusting Heart

The story of Noah's ark is not just a sweet story for children.
This is a foundational story to understand the heart and ways of God.

When I do not understand why an incident occurred, I have to step back and simply trust God.
While working in the hospice unit, I met an elderly man who had been married three times. His first two wives both died of breast cancer. Here he was again, sitting at the bedside of another cancer-ridden wife. I remember stamping my foot in the enclosed medication room and muttering, "It isn't fair."
I felt like a child stamping my foot, but this seemed so unfair. I couldn't comprehend it.

Can you imagine Noah with the specific directions to build the ark: use cypress wood of these dimensions, use pitch to coat it inside and out, bring two of each animal?
But eventually he had to realize, "There is no sail or rudder!"
How would you ever control this big boat and where would you end up?
Still, this man, blameless in the eyes of God, followed God's command and saved his entire family from a flood that covered the earth.

Lord, help me have a Noah-like heart, obeying You and trusting You.
Trust is a small word, but it has huge implications when it comes to our relationship with God.

Genesis 6:15

"This is how you are to build it: The ark is to be 450 feet long, 75 feet wide, and 45 feet high."

4

Share

Oh, merciful Lord,
I have so much.
I have more than I need.
Help me to see the needs of others so that I may share the love of God with them.
Help me not to become calloused in this career as I see pain daily and death all too often.
Remind me to keep empathy in the core of my heart.
Help me to put love before the task to be accomplished. I have deadlines to meet but I prefer to have Your love as my forerunner.

1 John 3:17

"If anyone has material possessions and sees a brother or sister in need but has no pity on them, how can the love of God be in that person?"

5

King Overall

The lab work is complete, the x-ray imaging report is back, and the physician is close to establishing a diagnosis. However, a physical is not complete without a history. That is why it is called an H&P, a history and physical.
We need to know the rest of the story.
Medical professionals must also be mindful of the unseen. Details such as how a person lives, his work patterns, habits of smoking, alcohol, and travels to foreign lands are all needed to put the puzzle together on what may be causing this illness.

God has many names.
Some of my favorites are Savior, Lamb of God, Good Shepherd, Bread of Life, Counselor, Prince of Peace, and My Father.
However, one that may be frequently forgotten is "Ancient of Days".
God knows your history, the number of hairs on your head, and if your mother's mother's mother was an alcoholic.
He knows all things from the beginning of times! I am in awe when I hear this name for Him.
You may come across it in an old hymnal.
Do not underestimate the power of this name.
He understands you better than you understand yourself because He knows your history from generation to generation.
As we focus on not what is seen but unseen, we are reminded that we worship a sovereign God.
He is king of a kingdom that is not of this world.

Daniel 7:13-14

"In my vision at night I looked, and there before me was one like a son of man, coming with the clouds of heaven. He approached the Ancient of Days and was led into his presence. He was given authority, glory and sovereign power; all nations and people of every language worshiped him. His dominion is an everlasting dominion that will not pass away, and his kingdom is one that will never be destroyed."

2 Corinthians 4:18

"So we fix our eyes on what is unseen. For what is seen is temporary, but what is unseen is eternal."

6

Love Like You

Oh, Gracious Creator of All Things, Heavenly Father!
Help me to love like You.
These are difficult times for those in need.
When someone is under my care there are financial burdens, relationship traumas,
family dynamic issues, as well as the physical issues that are paramount.
Help me to keep this in perspective when dealing with family members who are
stressed and burdened.
Please, Lord, help me to speak truth gracefully and help direct them to Your peace.
Help my love be evident in everything I do.

John 15:12-14

*"My command is this: Love each other as I have loved you. Greater love
has no one that this: to lay down one's life for one's friends. You are my
friends if you do what I command."*

7

Search My Heart

The internet is a great aid in looking up facts, symptoms, side effects of medication, and other details of medical care. What is the latest research on this rare medical complication I have encountered at work? What is a best practice for caring for this particular wound?
I can spend hours in research, seeking the best way to care for my patient.
I wonder, would I consider using the concordance in the Bible to look up a virtue I am struggling with in the midst of a personal disagreement?
Would I use the computer to look up all the verses in the Bible regarding forgiveness? Anger? Humility?
I know when I harbor feelings of resentment towards someone, my quality of caregiving decreases.
I am distracted and not focusing on what is important.
The Bible is complete.
It contains everything a person needs.
God's love letters to me answer my questions on what is truly important if I will take the time to look and refresh my mind with God's word.
Knowledge is good, but wisdom is better. God's word is eternal.

Jeremiah 17:10

"I the Lord search the heart and examine the mind, to reward each person according to their conduct, according to what their deeds deserve."

8

Praise Be to Him

Oh, merciful God.
Your name is to be praised and exalted above all things.
Help me to praise You even in the desperate circumstances that surround me.
What grieves me the most is when someone
is critically ill due to another person's actions.
A drunken driver, a gunshot wound, a new
baby born with heroin in his or her system.
My heart cries out for justice.
No matter where I am, my goal, Lord Jesus, is to praise You.
Some questions cannot be answered. I sigh in relief when
I remember that You do not change.
Your splendor stays the same no matter what circumstances I face.

Psalm 148:13

"Let them praise the name of the Lord, for His name alone is exalted; His splendor is above the earth and the Heavens."

9

Refined

The rings come off as I dress for my job as a nurse.
Keys, phone, badge, and lunch are the priority as I walk out the door.
Jewelry for me is a simple gold wedding ring.
Germs may harbor around diamond ring prongs, or worse yet, I could scratch
someone with my diamond wedding ring. As pretty as it is,
most days it is left behind in a drawer.
I have seen surgery canceled when a child was scratched accidentally
by a mom's wedding ring.
My gold wedding band is still perfectly round and minimally
scratched after many years of use.
The gold is not soft but was refined by fire.

In my walk to being a mature Christian, I know no one can be exempt from
hardship. Learning from mistakes and developing persistence may help grow
compassion, a needed ingredient in the recipe of any walk of life.

I pray my soul will be strong, shiny, and refined like gold.
This ring could be lost or stolen, but my faith will always be with me.
Thank you, Jesus, for this precious faith treasure.
You are my matchless treasure, and I am yours.

Isaiah 48:10

*"See, I have refined you, though not as silver; I have tested you in the furnace of
affliction."*

1 Peter 1:6-7

"In all this you greatly rejoice, though now for a little while you may have had to suffer grief in all kinds of trials. These have come so that the proven genuineness of your faith – of greater worth than gold, which perishes even though refined by fire – may result in praise, glory and honor when Jesus Christ is revealed."

Job 23:10

"But He knows the way that I take; when He has tested me, I will come forth as gold."

10

Knock

Lord, sometimes my heart is not in the proper place.
Sometimes I am hungry for the wrong things of this world.
Sometimes my desires cut short my empathy and my caring.
Lord, I knock on Your door for support.
You can give mightily if I believe and ask.
Let me open that door of belief and rekindle my heart to You.

Revelations 3:20

"Here I am! I stand at the door and knock. If anyone hears my voice and opens the door, I will come in and eat with that person, and they with Me."

11

The Cross

As you learn your anatomy in nursing school, you know the aorta is the biggest vessel in the body. There are 206 bones in the body, four chambers in the heart, two hemispheres in the brain, and three bones in the middle ear.
So many details you will need to draw upon as you help people with the complications of disease.
You need to know this stuff!
I learned firsthand…don't mess with the aorta!   There is trouble if the aorta is damaged in a car accident, if it out pouches with a weakness, or if it gets hardened with arthrosclerosis.

The cross is like the aorta when it comes to understanding God's love.
If you ever drift from God, lose interest, get mired down in the busyness of life, or lose heart, the best way back is by way of the cross. Jesus could have done it the easy way and just said, "All are forgiven."
Instead, He came down to earth to die on the cross because of His righteousness.

Jesus knows what it feels like to get discouraged and dismayed. When you feel like God forgot about you, come back to the foot of the cross.
There you will find a love that's divine.
Our just and righteous Lord understands. He, too, suffered.
Lord, thank You for dying on the cross for my sins.
Help me to value the eternal life You've given me in this perfect gift from the cross.

John 3:16

"For God so loved the world that He gave His one and only Son, that whoever believes in Him shall not perish but have eternal life."

12
Wonderful

Lord, Your love is wonderful.
Your love is amazing.
You made me and everything else in the universe.
Please let my words praise You when I inwardly groan with exhaustion.
As a caregiver, help me to realize that God lovingly created each patient.
They may not look or smell lovable, but God cares for all His creatures,
even the sparrows flying outside my window.
Help me to be merciful and gentle.
Help me to respect all that You have created.

Psalm 139:14

"I praise you because I am fearfully and wonderfully made; your works are wonderful, I know that full well."

13

Righteousness

When I am orienting a new nurse it is difficult to know where to start. You can't be too brief but you don't want to be too detailed, either. You might frighten this person away the first week on the job!
Protocol is important in many avenues of care, as it is not just what I "think" is best to do.
Where is the policy and procedure book or computer link?
It seems if a nurse falters, it is not because of the procedure, but more often a personal relationship dysfunction.
I try to be transparent and share part of my heart. I tell why I love nursing with the opportunities and challenges along the way.
However, some things are out of my control.

You can teach a person to ride a bike, but unless they enjoy riding the bike they most likely won't become proficient. Expertise comes with many days of trying it one way, and then failing or succeeding, and learning from those experiences.
Growing is the main thing.
We can't just stay the same. We are always learning and improving who we are; not just as a nurse but as a person. A unique person, one made to God's image.
No wonder we feel as if we have a hole in our hearts when He is not our center.
What is missing? If it is God, we need to mature and know He is the only way.

Orientation can last a week or six months, but our salvation is eternal.
Let us grow in the right direction. The ways of the world are temporary.
Let me grow closer to God, and in the process,
become more trained in righteousness.
Help me to know good from evil in a culture that may stray from what is right.

Hebrews 5:13-14

"Anyone who lives on milk, being still an infant, is not acquainted with the teaching about righteousness. But solid food is for the mature, who by constant use have trained themselves to distinguish good from evil."

14
Lord is My Guide

Lord, everyday there is a new challenge. A new time to prove my actions are
worthy of Your blessing.
I fall short often, in my thoughts and in what I do.
Help me remember that You will never leave me.
Please help me to encourage others.
Help me not to fear whatever the circumstances.
Lord, I know You have gone before me even before my workday started.

Deuteronomy 31:8

*"The Lord Himself goes before you and will be with you; He will never leave you
nor forsake you. Do not be afraid; do not be discouraged."*

15
The Lord is My Shepherd

If you are a nurse you will most likely have exposure to hospice care. People die. The entire 23rd Psalm is a beautiful prayer for those nearing death. When death occurs, the medial professionals may feel as if they have failed or worry about a lawsuit.

In Biblical times there were many shepherds and lambs to tend. We may compare it to the IT people now in our age of computer communication. Jesus called Himself the "Good Shepherd." People knew a good shepherd from a bad one, just as we know a good computer tech from an ineffective one. If a lamb was lost, the good shepherd would go look for him, risking the others that would be unattended.

When people's condition changes, I need to drop everything, get out of my schedule, and take the time to look into this complication that has arisen for this one particular person.

I want to be a good shepherd too, not just an on-time, orderly, and calm shepherd. Lord, help me to be effective in my work.

Guard over the patients that are left unattended while I help the one that is weak. Thank you for being my "Good Shepherd" and a wonderful example.

Psalm 23:1

"The Lord is my Shepherd, I lack nothing."

16

The Lord Heals

Disease and sickness surround me.
Most of the diseases and sickness are physical in nature.
However, many times they are matched by spiritual or psychological disease.
Help me to know that You are the greatest Healer.
You are the great physician as You designed every millimeter of the human body.
Lord, keep me strong. Heal me as I help to heal others.
I am in awe of Your wonder.

Exodus 15:26

*"He said, 'If you listen carefully to the Lord your God and do what is right in His
eyes, if you pay attention to His commands and keep all His decrees, I will not
bring on you any of the diseases I brought on the Egyptians, for I am the Lord,
who heals you.'"*

17

New Heart and New Spirit

God is in the business of changing people.
The stories I hear of people being radically changed often have a spiritual component.
Have you ever come across a person you consider to be just plain hard-hearted? If not, consider yourself fortunate! God can and does change people. Sometimes there is a praying mother or grandmother, a distraught wife, or a determined dad behind the scenes. One who does not give up on their loved one no matter what! They pray and pray and pray.
One day there is a change of heart.
The heart of stone turns to a heart of flesh.
One grandma told me she would kick her slippers under the bed when she went to bed. In the morning she would have to get on her knees to find her slippers and that was her reminder to pray. When you kneel in prayer you are serious about your prayer, and a strong faith must make Jesus smile.
Help me, Jesus, to protect my own heart. It is the source of my being. God created me, and He never intended my heart to be a heart of stone.
Protect me from evil and the evil one. Help me to develop persistence in my prayer for my loved one's salvation.
Thank You for Your promises, Lord. I cling to them again and again and know You are faithful.

Ezekiel 36:26

"I will give you a new heart and put a new spirit in you. I will remove from you your heart of stone and give you a heart of flesh."

18
The Lord's Healing Love

Lord, all around me people seem to be in trouble. Your promises of healing are
plainly stated in Your word.
You promise healing of body and soul.
Your love is refreshing and brings joy to my soul.
Your grace found me!
I am appreciative, Lord.

Psalm 107:19-21

*"Then they cried to the Lord in their trouble, and He saved them from their
distress. He sent out His word and healed them; He rescued them from the grave.
Let them give thanks to the Lord for His unfailing love and His wonderful deeds
for mankind."*

19

Pure Heart

Lord, help me to not lose my zest for life.
Help me to not be cynical or condescending. Keep my heart pure like Yours.
We know children smile many times more per day than adults.
Don't let me lose my child-like faith in You, my Father God.
Laughter can be the best medicine. Am I too analytical? Am I too scientific?
Help me to see things with a fresh outlook.
If I focus on what is best for the patient instead of considering the routine, I may
need to cut a new pathway.
Give me discernment and Your grace-filled ways to do what is best. Help me to
keep prayer in my heart day by day.

When I think of purity I think of new fallen white snow.
I pray You can create in me a pure heart,
one that is steadfast and does not easily falter, complain, or harbor self-pity.

Psalm 51:10

"Create in me a pure heart, Oh God, and renew a steadfast spirit within me"

20

Who Does God's Will?

Each day brings so many tasks, procedures, and meetings.
Unless it is documented you cannot even say it happened.
Check it off. Be accurate. Be on time. Smile. Enter. Delete. Save.
It seems there are not enough hours in the day.
I am exhausted.
I feel completely spent.
I want to be a part of your will, Lord. Can you use me?
I am willing.
When I am weak, Your strength shines through.
I rely on You, Lord!

Mark 3:35

"Whoever does God's will is my brother and sister and mother."

21
Jesus Wept

When I think families are being overly dramatic, I am reminded of Jesus weeping during His prayer time.
Even the Son of God had tears flowing down His cheek, worrying about what was to occur in the days ahead.
Tears can be healing. Tears can flow in times of sorrow or joy.

"Jesus wept."
What a simple verse to learn, but what a
powerful lesson in these two simple words!
Remembering this verse helps me to be more compassionate when family members display their emotions.

Help me to open my hands to what lies ahead in my day
instead of putting up my hands in protection.
I can follow Jesus' example as He was sinless.
Often times I miss the mark, but You forgive me
and strengthen me for the new day.
With prayer and reading the Bible I can know more of Your characteristics...like weeping when You were sad and weary. Your words in the Bible help me to be intimate with You.

John 11:35

"Jesus wept."

22

Good Medicine

Lord, help me to not only give out medicine, but to do it accurately and ethically.
Help me to not cause harm to anyone.
With all the time I take with medications,
this verse tells me that a cheerful heart is also important.
Who would ever want dried up bones? I see crushed spirits in every room I enter.
Let my eyes shine with cheer.
I cannot do this alone, but I know You can empower me.

Proverbs 17:22

"A cheerful heart is good medicine, but a crushed spirit dries up the bones."

23

Purity

What would a wedding be without music?
What would a dance recital be without a melody?
What would a birthday party be without the birthday song?
What would a mother, rocking her newborn to sleep in the still of the night, do
without a lullaby?

Music is important to me.
I am usually composed at funerals until the
music starts and then the tears begin to flow.
Music is known as the universal language.
On my way to work I choose to listen to Christian music on the radio or a
Christian CD.   Other times I sing a new song never before heard by mankind.
A simple way to praise God is to make up your own words, compose a poem, or
chant one thought
and sing it over and over again.
By singing I am simply seeking God's face, not making any requests.
By singing I am simply praising the One who is praiseworthy.

Psalm 96:1

"Sing to the Lord a new song."

24

From the Pit

I am sinful.
Within me there is a gossip, a slanderer, a liar, and a cheat.
I can be selfish, prideful, and lustful at times.
Even worse, I readily see these sins in others and want to pass judgment.
Who proclaimed me judge? No one!
More importantly, I need to confess my own sins.
I write my sins down in black ink and write over them sideways in red ink,
remembering how Jesus died for my sins and shed His blood for me.

Lord, ease the distress I feel and help me out of this pit of despair.
I do not want to feel blighted. I do not want to feel like withered grass.
My days vanish like a wisp of smoke if You are not with me.
Thank You for listening to me, a humble child of God.

Psalm 102:2-5

*"Do not hide your face from me when I am in distress. Turn your ear to me; when
I call, answer me quickly. For my days vanish like smoke; my bones burn like
glowing embers. My heart is blighted and withered like grass; I forget to eat my
food. In my distress I groan aloud and am reduced to skin and bones."*

25
Think about Such Things

Sometimes on my way home from work I will remember events and grumble,
"She actually said that?" "How could she have done such a thing?" "Why did
that have to happen?"
or "Why didn't he at least say he was sorry?"
On and on the record goes round and round in my head of what
'coulda, shoulda, woulda' happened.
Sometimes I think this makes me more tired than the actual work itself!
Lord, help me discipline my mind to focus on what is good. Eventually, my
thoughts will come out in my words, showing the world who I am as a person.
Focusing on what is good is my goal!
Instead of my grumbling, I will remember the positives.
"Thank you, Lord, for the person who held the door open for me as I walked into
the building."
"Lord, thank You for the lovely sunrise rays upon the green grass."
"Lord, thank you for the care-giving husband who sits next to his wife with
Alzheimer's."

Let me focus on what is noble and excellent.
If I have the eyes to behold it, I will find it.
Let me acknowledge good things by saying thank you to You, Lord.

Philippians 4:8

*"Finally, brothers and sisters, whatever is true, whatever is noble, whatever is
right, whatever is pure, whatever is lovely, whatever is admirable – if anything is
excellent or praiseworthy – think about such things."*

26

Grace and Weakness

Lord, it's by Your grace that we are saved.
Your grace is sufficient.
Colleagues, patients, and their families may become frustrated with me
if I am not up to par.
Strengthen me today in all my dealings with them.
Help me to take the burden You give me and learn from it.
There will be persecution, difficulties, and mistakes. Help me accept my
weaknesses and admit I am not perfect.
I will become strong in You, especially when I feel weak.

2 Corinthians 12:7-10

*"Or because of these surpassingly great revelations. Therefore, in order to keep
me from becoming conceited, I was given a thorn in my flesh, a messenger of
Satan, to torment me. Three times I pleaded with the Lord to take it away from
me. But He said to me, 'My grace is sufficient for you, for my power is made
perfect in weakness.' Therefore I will boast all the more gladly about my
weaknesses, so that Christ's power may rest on me. That is why, for Christ's sake,
I delight in weaknesses, in insults, in hardships, in persecutions, in difficulties.
For when I am weak, then I am strong."*

27
The Name of Jesus

I became more of an advocate for the name of Jesus as I studied other religions.
This verse in Philippians is quite specific. *Every* knee shall bow and *every* tongue
will acknowledge Jesus. Sometimes I only have energy and time for a one-word
prayer. When things are chaotic or confusing, I will whisper that word...Jesus.
If this one word can calm a storm or part a sea,
I want it uppermost in my thoughts.
Jesus, life gets complicated but Your love is simple.
Your love is a gift, a free gift, and I readily accept Your perfect gift.
Lord, help me to always say "yes" to the name of Jesus.

Philippians 2:9-11

*"Therefore God exalted Him to the highest place and gave Him the name that is
above every name, that at the name of Jesus every knee should bow, in Heaven
and on earth and under the earth, and every tongue acknowledge that Jesus Christ
is Lord to the glory of God the Father."*

28

Seasons Change

Lord, help me to remember that someday I may need the care of a caregiver.
Help me to make use of the health that You give me now, and please allow me the
empathy to take care of others as I would like to be treated.
If I am helping someone dress, help me to be gracious.
When I am helping someone eat, help me to be patient.
If my patient is worried or afraid, give me the words to calm them.

Our life path can take a detour when we least expect it. I may not always be
independent.
Grant me the opportunity to make the most of this season of health,
giving to others while preparing for the next season.

John 21:18

*"Very truly I tell you, when you were younger you dressed yourself and went
where you wanted; but when you are old you will stretch out your hands, and
someone else will dress you and lead you where you do not want to go."*

29
Caring for the Lonely

A friend of a friend was dying of HIV/AIDS, so I made a get well card for him.
I used a photo of a tree perched on the side of a mountain while a bird's nest rested in its branches.
Inside I copied the comforting verse from Matthew 6:26.
The nurses told us that when they found him, lifeless, he was holding a photo of his dog in one hand
and this greeting card in the other.
He died alone, with no one at his side.
I want to believe he knew God cares about the birds of the air and, more importantly, cares for him.
His parents were estranged from him. He had only a few friends.
But God cares for the poor of heart and the humble ones, and this accurately describes this man.
Lord, help me to be mindful and especially caring for those who are lonely.

Matthew 6:26

"Look at the birds of the air; they do not sow or reap or store away in barns, and yet your heavenly Father feeds them. Are you not much more valuable than they?"

30
With Everything

Lord, with everything I have and everything You want me to be, help me to love You.
Help that love overflow to the level of care You want me to show to my neighbor.
Who is my neighbor?
Do You consider the maintenance staff and the parking lot attendant in need of my love, too?
I need to first have love in my own heart and then allow that love to flow to others.
If my love-cup is empty inside it is difficult to offer a drink to one that is thirsty.
Only You can fill the void in my heart, Lord.
Sometimes I wonder if I am on the right path. Help me, Lord, not to doubt the path You have given to me, but to walk bravely with the strength only You can give. Help me see the people who need assistance.

Luke 10:27

"He answered, 'Love the Lord your God with all your heart and with all your soul and with all your strength and with all your mind; and, 'Love your neighbor as yourself.'"

31

Love Him

One day I found myself trying to explain how God loves us to a group of 8th graders in a children's Bible study program. It was hard for me to put it into words, so I used the analogy of a ferocious dog.
Yes! A ferocious dog!
A ferocious dog is persistent and keeps coming back for one more attack. A ferocious dog may be looked upon as a bad thing, but when you describe God's love as ferocious it is a good thing.
He comes to us through the back door, in a way we never expected.
He tries to get our attention through a calamity that may have happened or an illness in the family.
He allows us to fall down, hoping we will turn to Him.

Faith pleases God.
He pursues us as a bridegroom pursues his beloved. Ferocious love may just be the most unconventional but
perfect description of God's unrelenting love for us.
I pray God will pursue all my loved ones
ferociously so we can one day meet in heaven.
I cannot describe God's love completely, but for that hour, in that room, with the 8th graders, it was my heartfelt way to try and explain the wonders of God's love.
His love pursued me, and I am living proof of one changed. He loved me first.
I want to hand it off to the next generation.
I pray I can make a difference in the lives of my family for generations to come.

Deuteronomy 7:9

"Know therefore that the Lord your God is God; He is the faithful God, keeping his covenant of love to a thousand generations of those who love Him and keep His commandments."

32
Use Your Gifts

Sometimes I murmur, "If I can just get through this next shift."
Sometimes I don't feel like giving it 100%. Getting by seems enough.
I care for people in the hospital and then go home and care for my family.
At times I feel I don't have enough energy. Family members have even seen me
fall asleep with my uniform still on, a few minutes after I've walked through the
door.
At other times I am upset and unable to calm down. I drink chamomile tea trying
to slow down my motor that has been running at 100 miles per hour.
Lord, help me to not grumble. Who wants to hear my self-pity?
I prefer to use my gifts and run the race well.
This love that I have been given is like the frosting on a cake with some major
flaws. It covers the cracks and dents of the imperfect
cake so all anyone notices is the beauty of it.
I am forever grateful, Lord, for Your Love that covers my flaws. I want to do the
same for others.

1 Peter 4:8-10

*"Above all, love each other deeply, because love covers over a multitude of sins.
Offer hospitality to one another without grumbling. Each of you should use
whatever gift you have received to serve others, as faithful stewards of God's
grace in its various forms."*

33

All Things

Do you ever feel like you are working so hard, without a break for such long periods of time, that you are not sure you can get yourself up and do it all over again tomorrow?
Thoughts of vacations, spa treatments, and retirement start to dominate my brain.
This is when I grab my journal and talk it out by writing a note to Jesus.
Often I look back in the journal and notice all the
prayer requests that have been granted me.
I am encouraged that God has not forgotten me
and that His love is still surrounding me.
I know I can do all things through Christ who strengthens me.
I cannot do it on my own.
I am weak, but it seems that is the type of person God used in the Bible.
Moses stuttered. David had an affair.
Sarah laughed at God and Peter was impulsive.
Lord, help me to know I can rely on
You when I feel downhearted and discouraged.

Philippians 4:13

"I can do all this through Him who gives me strength."

34
My Shield

All around me are people trying to make me stumble.
It may be unintentional, but it is dangerous.
They say things to draw me into sinful behavior.
Help me to avoid these traps that surround me.
I say things that can harm others or lead them astray, as well.
I must be careful not to cause others to waver in their walk with God, either.
Unless I confess my sin I am not right with God. I want to be right with God, so I
will examine my heart and ask the Holy Spirit to see the sin
that may be hiding deep within.
The Holy Spirit is my helper. My helper is like a ball on a tether…
not conspicuous but there when I need help.
I have a shield to protect me from the arrows of sin that come my way.
I feel protected.
I like to speak the words from the Bible….
surely He will save me from the fowler's snare.

Psalm 91:3

"Surely He will save you from the fowler's snare and from the deadly pestilence."

35

Wisdom

On my way to and from work, I often play a game with myself.
As soon as my hands touch the steering wheel of my car, I am reminded to pray. I
ask God to keep my patients safe, to keep me from making a mistake, and from
saying an unkind or inappropriate word.
I pray that God will be my guide to help me walk on the path that He directs.
I know when I am left to my own devices things do not go as well as when Jesus
walks beside me and guides me.
I pray for my patients and my work, but I never forget my loved ones.
My spouse, children, grandchildren, sisters, brothers, friends, and neighbors are
uppermost in my heart,
and I pray that God will protect them. I take this praying responsibility seriously.
I may love my work, but I love my family more!

Prayer is as powerful as the laser beam in the radiology department,
and I would be crazy to try to live life without God's blessings.

Colossians 1:9

*"For this reason, since the day we heard about you, we have not stopped praying
for you. We continually ask God to fill you with the knowledge of His will through
all the wisdom and understanding that the Spirit gives."*

36
You Healed Me

Lord Jesus Christ, I need You.
I need You in all areas of my life.
I try to do well, yet I falter. I strive to do my best, but I fall short.
You healed me by dying on the cross for my sins. Help me to acknowledge that
and turn my life over to You.
Thank You for Your sacrifice.
Thank You for healing me.

Psalm 30:2

"Lord my God, I called to you for help, and you healed me."

37

True North

I can actually do more for my patients than is expected. I can go above and beyond what is considered routine, so I know I did my best. But the Bible tells me unless God builds the house, he who labors actually labors in vain. What I think may be the best thing to do could actually be the worst thing to do in a particular event. Dotting all the I's and crossing all the T's is not always enough. It is better to pray that God's will be done than to try and forge the trail single-handedly. I like to roll up my sleeves and do good, old-fashioned work, but if the focus is not on God it can be purposeless and ineffective. Lord, help me to stop and realize You are the creator. You are the potter. You told the seas where to stop and determined the height of the mountains. May Your will be done in all endeavors. You are my true north, and I will look for You as my morning star. Help me to pause in prayer as I begin my work.

Proverbs 19:21

"Many are the plans in a person's heart, but it is the Lord's purpose that prevails."

38

Chases Sickness Away

Lord Jesus, You extend a blessing over me that I don't deserve.
Although physically I am healthy, my spirit longs and needs You.
I am broken in many ways.
While sickness and death are part of the world today
You are the one to wash away sin and heal from the inside out.
You are my hope.
From Your eternal perspective, please chase the sickness away from me and
bring me into Your presence.
I do not deserve a thing. It is by Your grace I have breath. When I dream of
living a life of luxury, I will thank You for all the blessings I have already received
and appreciate each one.
I love living under Your wing of protection.

Deuteronomy 7:14-15

*"You will be blessed more than any other people; none of your men or women will
be childless, nor will any of your livestock be without young. The Lord will keep
you free from every disease. He will not inflict on you the horrible diseases you
knew in Egypt, but He will inflect them on all who hate You."*

39

With You, Love God

Caregivers of dementia patients are amazing people.
They care for their loved ones' personal needs. They give up
all sorts of things they used to enjoy.
They do not complain, and then the next day they do it all over again.
Helping those with memory impairment to eat, bathe, and dress is generally
tolerable, but when incontinence of bowel and bladder come into play,
it can be a difficult uphill road.
The person with dementia rarely says 'thank you' due to their impairment. It must
feel like an unappreciated job that goes on for years and years.

Amazing grace is what it is called.
Amazing love.
The caregiver loves the person as much, if not more, than when this all began.

Emmanuel, which means "God with you" is one of the many names of our Father
God. When you are weary and downtrodden who
do you turn to at the end of the day?

Jesus was a carpenter, and I wonder if He was not commissioned to make yokes
for the animals? I wonder if that was His most common work order? He spoke of
us being yoked to Him just as a young horse and a more experienced one would be
put together to get the field plowed.

Even if you cannot remember where any other verses are in the Bible, please know
where this verse is…it is the last verse in the book of Matthew.
It is easy to find and can be your 'thank you" from God.
He is saying, "Surely I am with you, loving and compassionate caregiver of your
demented spouse. You are not alone. I am there yoked with you. My yoke is
easy and my burden is light. I can help you. Surely I am with you to the very end
of the age."

Matthew 28:20
(The very last verse in the book of Matthew)

"And teaching them to obey everything I have commanded you.
And surely I am with you always, to the very end of the age."

40

Confess, Believe, and Be Saved

Lord, I have sinned.
I acknowledge that You, Lord Jesus, are my Savior. I need You above all things.
Help me profess with my words that You alone are worthy.
Guard my lips to say nothing that would displease You.
Help my faith in You be the cornerstone of my being.
Faith pleases You.
Help prepare my heart for You, Lord Jesus. I love you and believe in You truly.
Forgive my sins, and help me turn from them once and for all.
Help me to continue to help others carry their burdens.

I await the day I will see You face to face.
I look forward to the day when You will say,
"Well done, good and faithful servant."

Romans 10:9-11

"If you declare with your mouth, 'Jesus is Lord,' and believe in your heart that God raised Him from the dead, you will be saved. For it is with your heart that you believe and are justified, and it is with your mouth that you profess your faith and are saved. As Scripture says, 'anyone who believes in Him will never be put to shame.'"

ABOUT THE AUTHORS

D. Duane Engler is a son, husband, father of three, brother, and a friend. He loves the Lord and strives to work to Jesus in all he does, although often falling short.

As a professional educator and speaker D. Duane aims to help others live out Proverbs 4:26 as they consider the paths of their feet.

D. Duane resides in Edina, Minnesota, where he is working on his next book.

Marlene Graeve is a registered nurse with a Bachelor's Degree in business management. She has worked in pediatrics, assisted living and long term care, home health care, dementia units, and hospice inpatient care. She has earned certifications in gerontological nursing, hospice, and palliative care. She is presently employed at Superior Home Health Care in Lakeville, Minnesota.

Marlene is married, has 3 grown children, and 7 grandchildren. Marlene lives in Minneapolis and loves to vacation in Scottsdale, Arizona. She published the article "The Dementia Dozen: 12 tips for Alzheimer's Disease Caregivers" in Minnesota Health Care News Magazine.

Author's Section on Prayer and the 40 Prayers™ Series:

What is Christian prayer?

Prayer is communication with God. Communicating with Him from our place of weakness, surrender, and vulnerability so He would work in our lives, strengthening us for the tasks He has called us to do. Prayer is asking Him for guidance and skills that would allow us to honor Him more. Prayer is thanksgiving,

Prayer has been defined as an utterance, fervent request, entreaty, devout petition, praise, thanks, beseech, or crave. While the Internet provides many definitions of prayer, let's review vital points about prayer from a Christian perspective.

Is Christian prayer cross-cultural?

Christian prayer is cross-cultural and universal. God put the need for prayer in everyone's heart. Open Christian prayer is easier is some countries than others. Prayer to Jesus Chris is: (1) open and non-restricted, (2) monitored, (3) hostile, or (4) restricted depending on the country you live in or visit.

A Christian organization (The Voice of the Martyrs at www.persecution.com) defines these categories:

"Monitored areas are being closely monitored by some Christian organizations because of a trend toward increased Christian persecution. Hostile includes nations or large areas of nations where governments consistently attempt to provide protection for the Christian populations but where Christians are routinely persecuted by family friends, neighbors or political groups because of their witness. Restricted includes countries where government-sanctioned circumstances or anti-

Christian laws lead to Christians being harassed, imprisoned, killed or deprived of possessions or liberties because of their witnesses. This includes countries where government policy or practice prevents Christians from obtaining Bibles or other Christian literature."

The "God need" that is in our heart can only be filled by Him. Regardless of where you are or what country you are in, God knows your prayers even when prayer is not spoken out loud.

Who should pray?

Everyone. Christ calls us to pray to Him in all things for He is the way, the truth, and the life. No one comes to the Father except through Him. Start as early as possible praying with young children. The evil one knows he can tempt young children so you must start prayer early. You can even pray for children you want to have or the child that is in the womb.

Does God answer every prayer?

Pray and meditate on these verses regarding answered prayer:

1 John 5:14-15 *"That is the confidence we have in approaching God: that if we ask anything according to his will, He hears us. And if we know that He hears us – whatever we ask – we know that we have what we asked of him." NIV*

John 15:16 *"You did not choose me, but I chose you and appointed you so that you might go and bear fruit – fruit that will last – and so that whatever you ask in my name the Father will give you." NIV*

Matthew 7:7 *"Ask and it will be given to you; seek and you will find; knock and the door will be opened to you." NIV*

Romans 8:28 *"And we know that in all things God works for the good of those who love him, who have been called according to his purpose." NIV*

Isaiah 59:2 *"But your iniquities have separated you from your God; your sins have hidden His face from you, so that He will not hear."* NIV

If we go to God, but we are not in a right place with Him, what shall we do?

Ask God to prepare your heart to receive His Word. Read your Bible. Confess your sins. Ask a pastor or friend to seek direction by praying with them to God.

Where and when can we pray?

Anywhere and anytime. You do not need to close your eyes or be on your knees. On the other hand, you can close your eyes throughout your prayer and spend the entire time on your knees. Prayer happens in your heart and your mind. Keep in constant communication with him formally each morning or night and informally throughout the day. He is always there waiting for you.

What should we pray about?

Anything. Talk to Jesus as you would a friend. Tell Him what is on your mind, what you are concerned about, what you need help with. Thank Him and honor Him every time you pray. Ask Him for guidance and direction. Pray for your family and loved ones. Pray for people you do not even know by name. Pray for things big and small.

If God has full control and knows how things will end up, why then do we still pray?

We pray because He told us to do it. In Matthew 7:7, we are told to ask, seek, and knock. It's that simple.

Matthew 7:7 *"Ask and it will be given to you; seek and you will find; knock and the door will be opened to you."* NIV

How should we pray?

Many people who pray use the acronym "ACTS". ACTS stands for Adoration, Confession, Thanksgiving, and Supplication (which is a way of asking God for something). Do not worry if you are not sure which category your prayer fits in to or the full meaning of supplication. The reality is that God honors any sincere prayer.

As I am not an English major please forgive any grammatical or syntax errors in the prayers. When you pray, God does not care about the grammar or structure of your prayer. He just wants your heart; please give it to Him.

What type of application can you take from the 40 Prayers™ Series?

Application questions surrounding prayers and Bible verses are the most fun as it convicts my soul. Conviction draws me closer to the peace of walking with Jesus Christ. Consider these questions when you pray and read Bible verses:

1. What did this scripture mean when it was written?
An application Bible may be helpful – you can buy online or in any Christian bookstore.

2. What does this scripture mean for me today?
Reflect on what comes to your mind or what you are convicted by the Holy Spirit.

3. How can I apply this scripture to my life?
What specifically is happening in your life where this scripture fits?

4. What should I start doing, stop doing, or change?
Is there anyone who God has put on my heart that I should share this with?

If you need additional prayer, help, or assistance where should you go or whom should you contact?

Your local church or a trusted ministry to your specific need is a good place to start for help and support. The issues you face will benefit greatly from prayer. At times greater professional, medical, pastoral, or other support may be needed. Make sure you honor and respect your body, and do not be afraid to ask for help,

Why the 40 Prayers™ Series?

The 40 Prayers™ Series is a simple focus of prayer and action. The format is a topic, heartfelt prayer, and supporting verse. The intention is to make the books easy to access and read, efficient to pray for anyone, anywhere, and anytime, and filled with meaningful application with a biblical grounding in Christ.

What is the focus of the 40 Prayers™ Series Ministry?

1. Spark a revival in the lives of people through prayer to Jesus Christ
2. Reach others with the message of Christ's redeeming sacrifice of dying on the cross for our sins
3. Explain how to be productive, intentional, and resourceful with the gifts God has given us
4. Understand the need for prayer in our world

40 Prayers™ Series was started after numerous prayers on direction and application of God's truth in our life and the reality of God's sovereignty. Forty (40) is significant in the Bible as a number that means complete or completion. With these prayers my hope is that you would begin, develop, or enhance your relationship with Jesus Christ.

With the desire to leave a legacy of prayer for my family and children, I decided to retain my prayers for them in a written format. When a friend suggested I memorialize these prayers, I decided to publish them. After my death, my children will realize how important prayer was in their father's life. Hopefully, more than my immediate family will benefit from this series. My prayer is that these books would inspire you to pray, to grasp God's unconditional love and underserving grace, to bring people to accept Jesus Christ as their Savior, and to encourage and comfort others in need.

Many times in speaking with people we say we will pray for them or we write this in a greeting card. We end up neglecting that prayer time because we forget or are too busy. The 40 Prayers™ Series is something tangible you can send a friend or family member during life's needs, challenges, and celebrations, always keeping the focus on prayer.

I see a need for spiritual revival in our hearts, families, communities, and our world. Revival starts with prayer. As God as our sovereign Lord, if enough people reach out to Him in prayer, who knows what the outcomes could be. But He knows!

What can you do to support the 40 Prayers™ Series?

If you feel compelled, write a review where you purchased the book or recommend the 40 Prayer Series to others. That would be very gracious. You can bless one of your friends or family members with a copy. The book may bring him or her one step closer to accepting Christ as Savior.

We appreciate your support and fellowship through this prayer ministry. If you are feeling led to translate a book into another language, please let me know as we are in need of translators to reach others around the world. If you have ideas to benefit others through the 40 Prayers Series ministry or to reach more people, please let us know.

Let's rock the world with prayer!

May you live your life as a prayer honoring Christ Jesus in everything you do.
To our precious Lord Jesus Christ is the glory!

Many blessings,

D. Duane Engler

James 1:2-12

"Consider it pure joy, my brothers and sisters, whenever you face trials of many kinds, ³ because you know that the testing of your faith produces

perseverance. *Let perseverance finish its work so that you may be mature and complete, not lacking anything. If any of you lacks wisdom, you should ask God, who gives generously to all without finding fault, and it will be given to you. But when you ask, you must believe and not doubt, because the one who doubts is like a wave of the sea, blown and tossed by the wind. That person should not expect to receive anything from the Lord. Such a person is double-minded and unstable in all they do.*

Believers in humble circumstances ought to take pride in their high position. But the rich should take pride in their humiliation—since they will pass away like a wild flower. For the sun rises with scorching heat and withers the plant; its blossom falls and its beauty is destroyed. In the same way, the rich will fade away even while they go about their business.

Blessed is the one who perseveres under trial because, having stood the test, that person will receive the crown of life that the Lord has promised to those who love him." NIV

Made in the USA
Middletown, DE
24 May 2016